Your Hearts,
Your Scars

Your Hearts, Your Scars

ADINA TALVE-GOODMAN

EDITED BY
*Sarika Talve-Goodman
and Hannah Tinti*

BELLEVUE LITERARY PRESS
New York

First published in the United States in 2023
by Bellevue Literary Press, New York

For information, contact:
Bellevue Literary Press
90 Broad Street
Suite 2100
New York, NY 10004
www.blpress.org

© 2023 by the Estate of Adina Talve-Goodman

An earlier version of "I Must Have Been That Man" appeared in
Bellevue Literary Review.

"Sue Me" from *Guys and Dolls*
By Frank Loesser
© 1950 (Renewed) FRANK MUSIC CORP.
All Rights Reserved
Reprinted by Permission of Hal Leonard LLC

Library of Congress Cataloging-in-Publication Data
Names: Talve-Goodman, Adina, author. | Talve-Goodman, Sarika, editor,
    author of introduction. | Tinti, Hannah, editor, author of afterword.
Title: Your hearts, your scars / Adina Talve-Goodman ;
    edited by Sarika Talve-Goodman and Hannah Tinti.
Description: First edition. | New York : Bellevue Literary Press, 2023.
Identifiers: LCCN 2022020498 | ISBN 9781954276055 (paperback) | ISBN
    9781954276062 (ebook)
Subjects: LCSH: Talve-Goodman, Adina. | Heart--Transplantation--
    Patients--Biography. | Congenital heart disease--Patients--Biography. |
    Cancer--Patients--Biography.
Classification: LCC RD598.35.T7 T35 2023 | DDC 617.4/120592--dc23/
    eng/20220629
LC record available at https://lccn.loc.gov/20220204

Bellevue Literary Press would like to thank all its generous donors—individuals and
foundations—for their support.

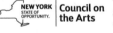 This publication is made possible by the New York
State Council on the Arts with the support of the Office
of the Governor and the New York State Legislature.

NATIONAL ENDOWMENT ARTS
arts.gov
This project is supported in part by an award from the National
Endowment for the Arts.

Book design and composition by Mulberry Tree Press, Inc.

Bellevue Literary Press is committed to ecological stewardship in our book
production practices, working to reduce our impact on the natural environment.

♾ This book is printed on acid-free paper.

Manufactured in the United States of America.

First Edition

10 9 8 7 6 5 4 3 2 1

paperback ISBN: 978-1-954276-05-5

ebook ISBN: 978-1-954276-06-2

For the very first time, the very first time,
I realized the fabulous extent of my luck: I could,
I *could*, if I kept the faith, transform my sorrow
into life and joy. I might live in pain and sorrow
forever, but, if I kept the faith, I could do for
others what I felt had not been done for me, and
if I could do that, if I could give, I could live.

—James Baldwin,
Tell Me How Long the Train's Been Gone

Contents

About Adina

MORE THAN THREE years after her death, it is still hard for me to read her words. I am grateful they live on, on the page, just as I am grateful for our text messages and emails and voice mails that now live somewhere in the cloud, even though revisiting any of it is painful. Adina and I became friends at six years old, and we were entwined ever since.

If you didn't know Adina, I can try to tell you about her.

She was brilliant and full of light. Her love for all of us was deep and unfiltered. She loved pretty shoes, even though all of them gave her blisters. She loved babies and McFlurry ice cream, and glitter. She loved little Italian restaurants and the movie *Moonstruck* and those sesame shrimp dumplings from Grand Sichuan. She made cup after cup of tea. She was the lead in the school play. She went to clown school and shined there.

Adina admired Audre Lorde and bell hooks and Maggie Nelson and the poet Jack Gilbert. She loved dance parties and pie and whiskey and cemeteries. She could eat so much lobster, much more than you'd expect. She hated onions and anyone who mistreated anyone she loved and this one girl from high school who still came to school one day even though she had bronchitis. She gave away cash to anyone who asked her for it. She loved boys with nice hands and retelling old stories with new and questionably true details. She sang loudly and off-key.

She was an excellent friend. When she passed, many people told me how lucky I was to have had a friend like her. They told me some people go through their lives never meeting anyone like that. At the time it felt meaningless, almost rude, but now I am starting to understand what they meant. You came to her in your highs and lows, in your quiet times and moments of celebration, and she was down for it all. Around her I laughed the hardest and cried the hardest. She fiercely reminded us how much we were loved.

Adina made everyone laugh. Sometimes if I say "Gina Lollobrigida" really fast, I can still hear her funny voice in my head. She would come and sit in the front row at my comedy shows. She referred to herself as "Stan"—a reference to an Eminem song about an unhinged fan. We'd often joke about who would die first and insisted on making a pact that whoever outlived the other had to name their firstborn after the deceased. She had impeccable timing. She told me she was being listed for a heart transplant at a hamburger restaurant called The Fatted Calf.

As time passes, I try to find a way to remember her apart from the overwhelming grief. I'll see a pretty pair of shoes or *Moonstruck* will be on TV. I'll hear a song she used to dance to, or someone will tell a joke about duck food, a joke I heard her tell one hundred times. I'll think, What a miraculous woman I have known.

Her words speak volumes, but this is all to give you the in-between. To trace why the pain remains.

—Jo Firestone

Your Hearts,
Your Scars

Introduction

ADINA CHAYA TALVE-GOODMAN, z"l (of blessed memory), wanted her first book to be a short and very good collection of creative nonfiction essays. The essays would be part narrative, part critical theory, and in a strange, artful, and nonlinear way tell the story of receiving a heart transplant in 2006, at nineteen years old. The essays would draw from lifelong experiences with chronic illness, exploring themes of embodiment, suffering, difference, ethics, and the racial, gendered, and sexual politics of ill and well bodies. Adina's writing was beloved by those lucky enough to read it, for its original and crisp narrative voice, and qualities of sincerity, humor, unpretentious intelligence, compassion, and warmth.

Adina was working on these essays when she became unexpectedly ill in the summer of 2017 with a rare form of lymphoma caused by post-transplant

immunosuppressants, post-transplant lymphopro-
liferative disorder (PTLD). She died the following
winter, in January 2018, at thirty-one years old. The
doctors had told us, her family, that this would be
curable in six months, after a round of chemotherapy. She died six months later, after four horrible
rounds. Her death was sudden and unexpected.
None of us was prepared to live without her, and
she wasn't readying for death. We were all terrified
and in shock during that whole period, but we had
hope; we thought we had much more time.

Adina loved the passage used as the epigraph
in this book, from her favorite novel by the writer
that she had loved most since she was a teenager,
James Baldwin. She kept it above her many writing desks and lived by those words, giving herself
to others in large and small ways, transforming
sorrow into joy through acts of kindness, humor,
and creativity. Adina held many hearts in hers.
She knew how to be present with and accompany
others through suffering and joy. It felt like everyone who met her fell a little bit in love with her.
Knowing Adina well also meant knowing that

the medicalized history of her body and her lived experiences of difference—especially in relation to bodies unevenly marked as other or strange—were central to her writing and the beauty in how she lived.

Adina wouldn't share the history of her body with just anyone. Here are some of the significant medical events, so you have an idea. Adina was born with a single ventricle heart and pulmonary atresia. She also had a form of spina bifida that caused a lipomyelomeningocele, a fatty mass attached to the spinal cord (I can hear her imitate the surgeon saying she's "just lumpy"). She also had mondini dysplasia and was deaf in her right ear. At one day old, she received a Blalock-Taussig shunt, attaching her subclavian artery to her pulmonary artery. At six days, the doctors added a second shunt, bringing her oxygenation up to 70 percent. She came home on the first night of Hanukkah, at two weeks old, one of the many miracle stories about Adina our mother would tell. At four months old, she had an eleven-hour spinal surgery that untethered her spinal cord.

She had this surgery again at sixteen. At two and four years old, she had an open-heart procedure called a modified Fontan. She went into heart failure at age twelve and was listed for a transplant at seventeen. She waited two years and received a new heart on October 27, 2006, which she marked as her "tranniversary," a day she approached with tenderness and weight. She lived eleven years with a healthy heart, with no rejection, described by a cardiologist as "perky."

Adina took medical leave from the University of Iowa to undergo chemotherapy after finishing her first year in the MFA Nonfiction Writing Program. She had complicated feelings about MFAs and didn't want to leave her full life and friends in Brooklyn for Iowa City. She had been working for almost a decade as managing editor at *One Story* literary magazine. There Adina came of age and into herself as an editor and writer, in the uniquely loving, supportive, and creative environment built by the *One Story* family. A boost came from winning a prize and her first publication in *Bellevue Literary Review* in 2017, for the essay "I Must Have

Been That Man." The MFA would buy her time to focus on her own work. In her brief time in Iowa, Adina found her beloved teacher and mentor Linda Bolton, z"l. Adina and Linda were beginning work together around critical intersections of embodied difference, race, illness and disability, ethics, suffering, and transformation, and would have done much more with more time.

The process of making this book has been raw and slow, a collaboration among people who love her and know her work—our family, the *One Story* team Adina worked closely with (Hannah Tinti, Patrick Ryan, Maribeth Batcha), and her dearest friend, Jo Firestone. We've stayed as close and true to her work as possible, honoring every fragment, every draft, every word. Some of the essays were drafts that she prepared for workshops and readings at Iowa. Others were in multiple versions—she often wrote this way, over long periods of time—and she likely would've returned to them, or let them go and written new pieces. At Iowa, she was moving toward a hybrid direction of creative nonfiction and critical theory.

"Your Heart, Your Scars, Zombies," which is a first draft, captures this. A future book likely would have dealt with her experience with cancer, and—based on conversations she was having with her loved ones—added important critiques to the militarized discourses around cancer and failing profit-driven systems that perpetuate this horrible disease.

Adina was my younger sister by two years and my best friend. She was brilliant, beautiful, wise, and the absolute funniest. Our parents, who are rabbis, would often ask Adina to talk to people experiencing different illnesses or surgeries—especially children—and she always said yes. She was giving and open when it mattered, when it helped others, and her creative work is another expression of that. Adina would sometimes reference a mysterious, untraceable description of a second-century rabbi of the Talmud, Shimon bar Yochai, that he had "one eye laughing and one eye crying." She used this image to capture her writing as broken and full of light. As she grew into herself as an artist, she had many mentors, colleagues, and friends along the way who believed in the importance of sharing her work with a wide audience, for the alternate futures and intimacies between ill, differently abled, and othered bodies that her voice calls into being. Her writing brings depth to conversations about embodied suffering, injustice and oppression, spaces between illness and wellness, living and dying, and how bodies of difference are marked and read as other and survive, transforming sorrows into joy. She wrote into in-betweens—what she called crawl spaces, or moments of light and undoing—with the fullness, joy, and reverence of how she lived.

When Adina's cancer treatments were starting not to go well, she said to me with a sadness and softness that she hadn't even gotten to publish a book. Of course she would, I said—she had been through worse, and she could get through this, too. I couldn't face the possibility of living without her. I feel the same pain closing in my throat now, almost four years later, as we prepare to share her work. I wish I had responded differently in that moment of openness. Maybe we could have talked about what she wanted and worked on it together, the way we worked on most everything else. After she died, I spent months and months reading and organizing everything she ever wrote, from fairy tales as a teenager to her most recent polished work, most of which I'd read and responded to over so many years. I reread all of her favorite books and watched all of her favorite movies. Right before she died, when it was clear she wasn't coming home from the hospital, she said that she was sorry for everything she had written in her notebooks about us, her family, that she didn't mean any of it. I knew she was talking to me and hope this meant she felt peaceful in some way about the idea of my reading her notebooks. I read and reread decades' worth of them, transcribing passages that felt less like private thoughts and feelings and more like places where she was working things out for an audience. I put a small manuscript together of polished pieces, a few pieces that existed in many drafts, and ephemera from the notebooks and sent it to my parents, Jo, and *One Story*. Hannah expertly edited the many drafts of "Thank God for the Nights That Go Right" and

"Should You Hold Me Down" into single essays, using all of Adina's words. The rest of the pieces are as Adina wrote them, with the exception of small and easy editing decisions that I made based on the versions that were the most ready to be shared. This is a book made out of love and grief, by Adina and by us, and I've done my best to reach as much as possible for the book Adina talked about wanting to write, that she was slowly and methodically creating.

Even though it would be hard for Adina—an opinionated artist and critic—to have her work shared in unfinished form, she would probably soften to its being imperfect and fragmentary, a perfect gift to those who might need it. In the darkness of grief, we can only offer her unfinished work out of love, the way I know she would have when she was ready. I am endlessly grateful to Hannah Tinti for her care and skill as an editor; to the whole *One Story* team for their steadfast support; to our family; to all of Adina's friends and dear ones who stay connected to us and one another. Adina would probably be as gentle and generous about this book as she was with most everything and everyone in her life, giving it over to love, to us, whose hearts are bound up with hers, trusting whatever is carrying us through, and what will carry you.

—Sarika Talve-Goodman

I Must Have Been That Man

"I suspect there was some kind of fall," she said,
"even if it was just a little stumble."

—James Tate,
"I Must Have Been That Man"

O N A MONDAY NIGHT IN OCTOBER when
I was twenty, I walked home with a boy
from a party, drinking cheap whiskey and sharing
puffs of his cigarette. We stopped on the stairs
outside of my apartment and kissed. I asked if he
wanted to spend the night. This is healthy, I told
myself, this is college.

In my room, we laughed and shushed each
other, fumbling around with buttons and zippers
until he took off my shirt.

"What's this?" he said as he traced the scar
down the middle of my chest, his fingers lingering
on the keloids, the small, hardened lumps of scar

tissue that punctuated the already prominent pink line.

"I had a heart transplant," I said.

"When?"

"A year ago."

"Oh."

I waited for him to ask the usual questions: Why did you need it? Are you okay now? What about the donor?

"You have great boobs," he said.

After he fell asleep, I got out of bed and felt around in the dark for a shirt. I could only find his flannel, so I put it on like a robe and walked to the bathroom. I opened his shirt in front of the mirror and placed my fingers on each of the keloids, imagining I might be able to play my breastplate like an accordion, find the right note, and have the scar disappear.

Even after a year, the straight scar down my chest hadn't become a part of my landscape like the rest: the two scars on my back that frame my shoulders like wings, the scars on each rib that tan in the summer and look like scrapes in bark, and all the small ovals where suction tubes once were that could easily be birthmarks or sunspots. But the transplant scar remained surgical-looking and wouldn't blend or sink. It sat there, hanging just below my neck.

To the left of the scar, I could see the new heart beating beneath my skin. Some nights, shortly after the surgery, it beat so hard, I couldn't sleep. I would lie awake listening to its unfamiliar rhythm: bump-BUMP bump-BUMP. The new double pump song of perfection replacing the one wrong beat, a single ventricle, I had had before.

Sometimes I'd fall asleep and dream of people dancing in ballets with symphonies coming out of their mouths when I expected words. I didn't tell anyone about the dreams. I was afraid they'd say that maybe it was the donor, maybe the donor had danced.

I tried not to think about the donor much. I'd spent close to two years waiting, always wondering what the donor might mean, what might change in me. I'd seen kids lose themselves in their donors. They'd make websites dedicated to living the life their donor never got to finish. They'd talk about their donor as if they were friends. When I listed, my parents, both rabbis, told me a story from the Talmud about a rabbi who goes to visit three sick men and each time the rabbi asks, "Is your suffering dear to you?" "That's the whole story," they'd explain, "and it's the question that's important." I took it to mean this: When the time comes, will you be able to live without the heart defect that always made you special and strong? Will you be able to face wellness and normalcy? Will getting a good grade be as big of an accomplishment if you didn't have to study in the hospital to get it?

So, when the call came, I didn't ask where the heart was coming from or where it had been. And when I started dreaming in ballets, I didn't go looking for answers in my donor. Instead, I decided this must be how people with healthy hearts dream: in music and dancing, kicking off blankets and sheets in the middle of winter because my blood had never moved so fast through my veins and the warmth of it was almost unbearable.

After the surgery, the doctors said that it would take a year, a full year, for the heart to thaw and reach its capacity. Now, at almost a year, I stood in front of the mirror in a boy's shirt, wondering how long it was going to take until that new rhythm wouldn't keep me up at night. How long I would have to live with this new heart before it would feel like mine and I would forget the years I'd spent waiting, getting too close to death.

How many cigarettes I would have to smoke, how many boys I would take home to prove to myself, and the new heart, that this body was still my house.

Is your suffering dear to you?

No, I thought.

In the morning, I hid his cigarettes and made him toast and everything was funny again. We had headaches, we smelled like whiskey, and it was a Tuesday. He left for class, and I stayed home because I didn't have classes that day, just rehearsal for a play in the evening. He told me I should come find him later, before my rehearsal, he'd be at the library, and he'd be happy to help me learn my lines.

After he left, I showered, got dressed, gathered my books, and walked outside. It was October in St. Louis and not quite cold. There was a slight drizzle and even though I was wearing a raincoat, I could hear my mother's voice saying, "You're immunosuppressed; please take an umbrella." That's when I realized I was locked out.

The walk to campus wasn't long, fifteen minutes, and even though I had a car, I walked it almost every day. I liked to walk it alone. Before the transplant, fifteen minutes was impossible. The doctors explained it to me like this: "For you, in heart failure, a fifteen-minute walk is like a marathon and that's why sometimes you throw up at the end." Doctors often explained my illness to me using sports metaphors—as if, as a kid born with a single-ventricle heart, sports was a language I ever learned to speak.

I sat on my stoop and rubbed my head, regretting my decision to forgo a Tylenol. Both of my roommates were on campus, most likely with the boy from the night before. He was probably smoking a cigarette outside the library, not knowing the gift he had given me by not asking questions and treating my body like I hadn't been split down the middle and pieced back together. But now he knew that I walked around that campus with a perpetually broken chestplate and a very loud heart. And for that reason, I didn't want to see him again.

I walked instead toward a coffee shop. I kept to the side streets and little alleys because I felt as if I might cry, and if I did, I didn't want to run into anyone who might try to talk to me about it. Halfway down the street, I saw a man lying on the ground, his electric wheelchair fallen beside him in the dirt.

As I got closer, I recognized him. He rode around the Loop a lot and I remembered talking to him a few times when I would sit outside at the coffee shop. He always asked what I was reading, but he never seemed to remember that we'd

31

met before. Earlier that spring, he stopped by my table on a sunny day and said, "You're just lovely." I thanked him and I meant it, because on some days after the surgery, I would look down at my chest to make sure it wasn't bleeding, to make sure you couldn't see that underneath my shirt I had been stapled together and might one day do something clumsy, slip on the sidewalk, and come undone. I was put together fine (expertly, in fact), but something remained unhealed in me that spring and it comforted me to know the world hadn't noticed.

When I was close enough to speak to him, he propped himself on his elbow and adjusted his glasses.

"Well, hello," he said.

"Hi," I said.

"Walking in the rain, huh?"

"I locked myself out of my apartment," I said. "I'm on my way to the coffee shop."

"Oh, that's nice," he said as he tried to pull himself into a sitting position. He couldn't manage to sit, so he continued to prop himself from one elbow to the other. I set my bag down on the ground.

"Can I help?" I asked.

"Oh, it happens all the time," he said. "My chair doesn't work so good in the rain. I'm saving for a new one. It's lighter and it goes faster. You look familiar."

"We've met. Outside the coffee shop. I'm—"

"Oh, yes! You read a lot."

I blushed. "I'm a student." I've always been self-conscious of my reading, as if it betrays that I have stayed home for an embarrassing chunk of my life.

"You must be a good one," he said.

"I'm okay." There was a pause between us, and the rain picked up. "Can I help you get back in your chair?" I asked.

"Oh, no, no," he said. "I'll be just fine. I live right over there with my mother. I'll get up eventually, I just need a little time."

"Can I call her for you?" I asked.

"No, no. She's still at work. She'll be home in an hour."

"Well, maybe I can just turn the chair upright," I said.

"Ha!" he said. "Like to see you try!"

The chair was behind him and somehow I managed to turn it right side up, but it wasn't easy. I'm not sure how I did it and I don't think I could do it again. After, I sat down beside him to catch my breath. I was already wet, so I took off the hood of my raincoat.

"You are stronger than you look," he said.

We both laughed. "Do you want to try to get back in the chair?" I asked.

"Well, it looks like you're some kind of weight lifter so, yeah, let's try."

I hooked my arms underneath his shoulders and he pulled up on the wheelchair. On three, we both lifted, but the weight of his legs was too much. We fell back into the dirt. He was about six feet and over three hundred pounds, with everything from his waist down tethering him to the ground. I couldn't lift him, not even a little. I wrapped my arms as far as I could around him as he pulled up on the wheelchair, but the few inches he got off the ground were from his own effort. While we were struggling and sort of hugging like that, he asked me what I did.

"I'm a student," I repeated.

"But what do you study?"

I was a Women, Gender, and Sexuality Studies major, but the last time I had said that to a man, he'd replied, "Yeah, me, too," with a horrible wink.

"I study theater. I'm an actress," I said.

"Oh yeah? Yeah, I could see that. You're real pretty. I bet you're a good actress."

"I'm okay," I said again.

"Are you in anything right now?"

"I am. A comedy at my college."

We lifted again and from behind me I heard a gruff "Hey!" We fell and I turned to see a white pickup truck. The driver gave us the up-and-down and said to me, "You all right?" I looked around like maybe there was someone else in trouble. Then I realized what the truck driver must've seen: a tiny white girl struggling beneath the weight of a large black man on a side street in St. Louis.

"I'm fine," I said. "We were just trying to get him back in his chair."

The man's brow unfurrowed and, suddenly, he saw the electric wheelchair, as if it hadn't been there before. He parked his pickup in the middle of the street and climbed down to help. We tried to lift the man with just the two of us a few times but still couldn't manage to set him in the chair. Because the man was so tall, the seat of the wheelchair was high off the ground. And because of the rain, the chair had short-circuited, and the seat wouldn't lower.

"Wait here," the man with the truck said. "I'm working construction a block away. I'll get my guys."

He took off running down the alley, leaving his truck parked in the middle of the street. I sat down to wait beside the man, whose name I didn't know. The rain picked up and the dirt around us started turning to mud.

"You can go," the man said. "It's so nice of you to wait, but I'll be all right. It'll come back on, the chair, it always does."

My heart was pounding from trying to lift the man. I looked at him now, sitting propped against his chair, and couldn't find the words. I thought about unzipping my jacket, peeling off my high-necked shirt, and showing him my chest. Pointing to each and every scar, hoping this might act as our common language. Here, I would say, was a suction tube that stayed in for three days; here is where they do biopsies every six months now by taking little pieces of the heart out through my neck; here is where my muscles were cut when I was four years old for a repair that didn't work. I wanted to explain to him that I wasn't good at much, but I was good at waiting. How I had waited nearly two years for a heart, and a year ago, I had come so close to death that sometimes I worry the smell of it lingers on my body and maybe that's the reason I buy so many clothes and creams. So when

I said, "I'm happy to sit here with you," I meant it with all of my hearts.

The man with the truck returned with two more men. As the three men tried to lift the one man into his chair, the man being lifted told the Mexican man he was reading a book about the Mayans. He asked if the Mexican man was Mayan, and the Mexican man replied, "Not anymore."

There was a lot of tugging and pulling at the man's wet clothes to hoist him toward his seat. A lot of "One. Two. Three. LIFT." I turned away because his pants started to fall. It was humiliating and uncomfortable, but once he was in the chair, he thanked us and said he could handle it from there. He said we should all go, the rain was lighter now and he could wait until it stopped and the chair came back on, as it happened all the time. But the chair would not turn on and the men would not give up.

"No, no," one of the men said, "we'll carry you home." Then they all chanted "carry you home."

The chair was heavy, and the men had to stop to catch their breath several times. A man who owned a Chinese restaurant nearby had also joined us, and he held his yellow umbrella over the other men. They were like a parade now, a march, and I continued to walk beside them, not knowing why I was still there. I hadn't been able to help in a while.

When we reached his house, his mother opened the door. She's home from work, I thought; it must have been over an hour since I first sat down beside him in the dirt.

She thanked us all, adding, "You didn't have to carry him in the chair. The chair will come back on. It always does." I was ashamed then and I couldn't meet her eyes.

They lived on the second floor, with no elevator, and one of the construction workers asked how he would get up the stairs. "He does just fine," the mother said. She was fierce and we deserved it.

I shook the man's hand and he held mine a moment. "Good luck to you," he said.

My throat was tight and I could barely breathe—bump-BUMP bump-BUMP, it screamed. "I'm sure I'll see you around," I said.

"Oh, sure you will. I'm always around."

When his mother closed the door, the other men were peeking in to see him get up the stairs using only his arms. I was already in the street, walking back to where I had left my bag in the mud. The three construction workers and the man with the umbrella caught up to me. They were laughing about how they were like a bad joke: a black guy, a white guy, a Mexican, and a Chinese guy find a man in a wheelchair. . . . They patted one another on the back as we walked, saying how lucky that man was that I'd found him, how he would've been "shit up a creek" without me.

"I didn't do much," I said. One man held the umbrella for shelter, one man went for help and brought the two other men, who finally hoisted the man back into his chair and carried him home. All I really did was sit beside him and wait in the in-between.

The man with the truck asked if I needed a ride anywhere. I said, "No, thank you." The rain was lighter now and the coffee shop was only a few blocks away. He piled into the truck with the other two construction workers and they drove away. The man with the umbrella asked if he could walk with me so that I might stay dry. I said, "No, thank you." I was already wet. We parted ways and I sat back down in the mud and cried. Someone walked by and gave me a smile but didn't stop. College girls cry all the time.

When I walked into the coffee shop, I made a puddle of muddy water on the floor. I spotted a friend at a table in the corner and she waved me over.

"You look like you've been through a war," she said.

I took off my coat and realized my clothes were soaked through. I went to the bathroom to clean myself up.

I was shivering and there was mud all over my face and hands. I stood in front of the mirror and thought about going back to the man's apartment to apologize to him. I didn't know what I would say. We couldn't have left him there in the mud, I suppose, but I should have just listened to him and waited alongside him awhile. Nothing would've been fixed, not the chair or the man's body, and we wouldn't have talked about how we might try or the new features of his coming chair. We would've just sat together, side by side in the mud, talking about books and school, staring across some invisible river at ballets and marathons, able bodies and recognizable rhythms. And that alone might have been better than three men lifting his body into a stubborn and broken chair.

I turned on the faucet and waited for the water to warm.

It takes a year for the heart to thaw.

I washed my hands.

The chair will come back on, it always does.

I wet a paper towel and wiped the mud off my face. I stopped shivering and started to warm up. It happened so quickly: warming up from a healthy heart and fast-flowing blood. My cheeks were flushed and my clothes clung to my body. I looked in the mirror—flushed cheeks, big breasts, pink lips—a body that smoked cigarettes and drank whiskey on Monday nights and could still lift wheelchairs the next day. A body that now slept beside other hearts of the same beat and warmth. A body finally good enough to say "No, thank you" and no one would insist on carrying me home. I removed my shirt to wring it out in the sink. I traced my scar and looked at the quick rise and fall, the vibration in my chest—the raging, healthy heart.

Is your suffering dear to you?

Yes. A little bit, yes.

San Diego, 2001

WHEN I WAS FIFTEEN, I went on a week-long trip to San Diego, staffed with nurses for teenagers who'd had organ transplants. Most of them kidneys, a few livers, no lungs, and two hearts. Lungs, I'd heard, were the most difficult of all. Lungs were the transplants you sometimes measured your own gratitude against. It could be worse; you could need lungs. The girl waiting on lungs and I were the only two teens on the trip with all our own organs.

In the mornings, the nurses served us bacon and we ate fast food most of the day. Each night, there was a bonfire on the beach and one of the hearts, a boy from Michigan, insisted we make a circle, hold hands, and pray. It was not a religious trip, but they all agreed it was a good idea. They bowed their heads, nurses and recipients together, and thanked Jesus for the organs he had given them. There was no mention of donors, living or dead. I sat just outside the circle, eating granola bars my mother had packed for me and thinking that Jesus must be full of kidneys. On the second night, a girl sat down behind me in the sand and whispered, "Is you Jewish?" I could not see her face. "I think you are," she said. And then: "It's okay, I won't tell." She had a new liver; she said she got it from her dad.

Before the bonfires and prayers, the boy from Michigan would play soccer with his shirt off on the beach. He had blue eyes, round cheeks, and a good-looking scar. Flat, delicate, straight down between his pecs, catching sun on his tanned body, as if it were something natural to him, as if it belonged. We all noticed its beauty, even the nurses. It's a beautiful scar, we said. I overheard the nurses say his chipmunk cheeks would go down soon; in a few months, he would be weaned off of prednisone. His transplant had been recent, within the year. Within the year, they said, sighing, and he plays soccer every day. He held the ball between his ankles and kicked it up behind him to a boy with a new kidney who wasn't ready.

One night, after prayer, the girl waiting on lungs and the boy with the beautiful heart scar went walking. I watched them go, holding hands on the edge of waves in moonlight with their shoes off. They didn't get far, hearts and lungs— she probably couldn't take the walk. Later, all the girls gathered in one of the hotel rooms to listen as she sat perched cross-legged on a twin bed, holding a pillow and recounting how he had kissed her with tongue. She'd had better. He was a little boring, she said; they talked mostly about how much he loved soccer—but his eyes, and his scar, sure were beautiful. I wondered if she could tell the difference between kissing the boy from Michigan and boys without displaced hearts. Could she taste it? Did she stroke his swollen pink cheeks? And when they paused so that she could catch her breath, did she touch his scar? Was it as soft as it looked? She kept kissing him after prayers each night and then holding court in the hotel room after. On the fifth night, my friend with a liver from her father whispered, "I would've blown that boy already." She was tired of all the talk, kissing, and beaches. She would've blown that boy from Michigan—wouldn't I? "Probably not," I said. She was surprised. Most of the Jews she knew were sluts, she said.

On the walk back to our rooms, my friend with the liver from her father went on about how much she loved blow jobs. Giving them, she giggled, watching the boys' faces as they came in her mouth. I asked how she could see their faces in that moment. Didn't she have to look elsewhere—at their crotch, or their thighs, by necessity? "After," she corrected. One boy, she told me, cried. Her boyfriend loved them most of all.

"Most of all?"

"Hands and mouth stuff," she said.

She told me she liked to swallow and then showed me her technique. She licked all around her mouth, beyond her lips, as far as her stubby tongue would reach just below her nose. Then she folded the skin she had wetted and her lips over

47

her teeth and ran the spitty mouth pocket up and down the side of her left arm. "Just like that," she said. "They all love it just like that." She wiped her mouth and smiled. I asked why she liked to swallow, and she said she liked the taste of cum.

"What's it like?"

"7UP and salt," she said.

We sat outside her room together, talking blow jobs and cum for what felt like a long time, our backs pressed up against the cool stucco wall of the hotel. Eventually we were quiet enough to hear the waves from the Pacific. She told me this trip was the first time she'd seen the ocean—was it mine? No, I'd seen oceans; I'd even been to San Diego before. Why was I here? She wanted to know.

"I might need a heart transplant," I said. A social worker had thought that meeting other transplant kids might help normalize the experience, make me feel less afraid.

"What're you afraid of?" she asked.

"Most things," I said. Then I asked her about her father, about having a piece of his liver inside her. She said she didn't think about it much but that in the months that followed the transplant, her favorite thing to do was go out to diners with her dad. They'd sit in a booth, their upside-down Y scars facing each other beneath their shirts, eating all the foods she hadn't been able to digest before. Eating and swallowing anything she wanted, anything she craved.

♥

THE NEXT DAY WE VISITED SeaWorld. It was humid and the girl waiting on lungs was having trouble taking deep breaths. I volunteered to push her and her small oxygen tank in a wheelchair around the park. We went slowly, away from the group of healthy teens with healthy organs, along the edge of the stingray pool. Other visitors were reaching in and touching the tops of the stingrays, pulling their hands out quickly once they found one. The girl waiting on lungs said she'd like to touch a ray. I offered my arm to help her out of

49

the chair and she leaned into me. She smelled like peaches and vanilla lotion. I wondered if she leaned on the boy from Michigan as they walked each night. Did he know that she leaned this way out of necessity?

We sat on the brick edge of the pool and as she bent down to touch a stingray, the tubing from her tank went taut and she pulled back. "Sometimes I forget it's there." She laughed. She removed the oxygen from her nose and took a deep, shuddering breath. I thought for a moment she might dive in to swim with the rays. She didn't, though. She reached her hand down into the water and ran her fingers over one of their backs. "It's rough!" she squeaked. "Feel it."

On top of the brick were mosaics of leaping, happy sea creatures. The pool was shallow, not very big. The stingrays crowded into the center and the ones on the edge raced inward, trying to avoid human touch.

"You look pale," she said. "Want a hit of oxygen?"

"No, thank you," I said. "That doesn't really work for me."

"I guess not," she said.

I reached my hand in. The water was warm, and I grazed the top of a ray close to me. The girl waiting on lungs was right—the skin of the ray was rough and cool to the touch, much colder than the water around it. It swam away, but I kept my hand in the lukewarm pool, in case it came back to sting me or in case I was wrong and they loved the touch.

"Have you done Make-A-Wish yet?" the girl waiting on lungs asked as she put her oxygen back in her nose and slid into the wheelchair. I pulled my hand out of the water.

"No," I said. "I don't think I qualify."

"You totally do!" she said. "You totally do. If you qualify for a heart transplant, you totally qualify for Make-A-Wish. You should do it. I went on a shopping spree." She held up her arm to show me the silver bracelet with a large Tiffany-style heart

51

pendant dangling from the center, knocking on her small bones. "I got this," she said.

I retook my position behind the chair and pushed us toward an indoor exhibit. She told me about all the wishes that had been made on that trip. She spoke softly, as if they were secrets, or maybe because of the humidity, because it made it just the slightest bit more difficult for her to breathe. I leaned on the back of the chair so I could hear her as I pushed us along. The boy who had gotten a kidney from his brother wished to ride in a race car with his favorite NASCAR driver—but they wouldn't let him drive or go over sixty. The girl from rural Kansas who got a liver from a neighbor wished to go on a beach vacation with her family in Los Angeles. My friend with a liver from her father also wished for a shopping spree. "Shopping is a popular wish," the girl waiting on lungs said. "What would you wish for?"

We reached the World of Fishes exhibit and a woman wearing a pink fanny pack rushed to open the door for us. She looked down at the girl waiting on lungs and her small oxygen tank and rubbed my back as I rolled us through the door. "What a good girl you are," she whispered in my ear. We both thanked her. All I could see was blue as my eyes adjusted from the sun. Then the aquarium, the fish swimming inside. I rolled us close enough to reach out and touch the glass. The girl waiting on lungs reached first and tapped, the large heart swinging from her wrist. "What would you wish for?" she asked again.

"I've never thought about it," I said.

"You should," she said. "You have to wish before you're eighteen. After that, you don't qualify anymore."

I smiled. After eighteen, you're dying like the rest of the world. After eighteen, you're not so tragic.

"I'll keep that in mind," I said.

♥

ON THE LAST NIGHT, we didn't go to the beach. We walked along the boardwalk and had cash to pick our own food. I was relieved and, in my relief, felt a kind of ecstasy and hunger. I chose Greek food and the boy from Michigan noticed.

"You like Greek food?" he asked.

My family is Sephardic, so I heard it as "Jew food."

"Only a little," I said. "Mostly I like cheeseburgers."

"Me, too," he said. "My donor, though, he liked Greek food, so I try to eat it sometimes."

My donor: he. A boy, a dead boy, a dead boy who had liked Greek food. We stood in line side by side at the Greek place, so close that I could feel the boy from Michigan's soft blond arm hair brush mine. I wanted to ask how he had come to this ritual of eating food he disliked to please his heart. Could he feel the heart open and reconstitute into a boy with a mouth, a gut, a taste for Greek food? And why Greek food—what else do you know about the boy who died this year? Do you have other rituals like this one—away from bonfires, away from Jesus, alone? But he asked me instead why I did not say grace before we ate, why I did not join his prayer circle at night.

"I still have all my organs," I said.

He laughed. There was some relief, maybe, in acknowledging that I did not know what it felt like to carry the weight of dead donors. I did not yet have a living altar inside my body, did not feel the need to present it with something like Greek food. He asked me why, what was I waiting for.

To get sick enough, I told him.

He didn't understand. The boy from Michigan's transplant had been quick. A virus, he said, one whose name he never needed to learn. He'd gotten sick and received a new heart all in three weeks. He had never been in the hospital prior to the virus, had never had surgery before, had never made a wish. His scar was so beautiful, smooth and pristine, because it was made with better tools than mine and was his first. He was good at soccer, much better than the other boys on the trip, because he had played before. On a team, in a league, and he was practicing each day to get back to his life. He had been a healthy boy and the way he said "my donor, he," the way he stared bewildered at the menu on the wall behind the counter, the way he asked me, "What does *tzatziki* mean?" made me want to tell him I was so sorry for his loss.

The Condition of My
Transplanted Heart Is
One of Remembering

THE HEART CAME FROM SOMEWHERE in the
Midwest by plane to St. Louis Children's
Hospital during game five of the 2006 World
Series between the St. Louis Cardinals and the
Detroit Tigers. My mother heard cheers as the
surgeon stepped off the elevator with the cooler
containing the organ. She took a picture of the
surgeon and the cooler in the same moment that
Adam Wainwright threw the final pitch, a strike,
to Brandon Inge and the Cardinals became
champions. In the picture, the surgeon is smil-
ing. The cooler containing the organ is navy blue;
the surgeon holds it with one hand. Years after
the transplant, I find the photo on my mother's phone while trying to help her clear space

for more memory. She asks me to leave it there because she sometimes likes to look at it. I zoom in on the cooler—it is the closest I've ever come to seeing the heart now inside my chest or a picture of the donor.

My own heart I've seen. After it was taken out, I asked if I could bring it home with me. It was an "unusual" request, one the hospital had never fulfilled before. My cardiologist asked if it was a Jewish thing. My parents are rabbis and they both said no, it's not a Jewish thing to take your organs home with you. All I could say was that I wanted it, it had been mine, and I didn't want it to be thrown away. They released it to me in an urn through a funeral parlor as my own "remains." I suppose it does remain, in a way, as evidence of the great event. I now have two hearts in my possession: one inside, and one out, in an urn. The process of getting my heart released took a few weeks. I went to the hospital for a checkup around Thanksgiving, and my doctor presented me with a square wooden box. It was the cheapest urn, my mother said.

My family doesn't usually do much for Thanksgiving. But the year of the transplant, our gratitude was overwhelming, so we made about seven kinds of pie and then opened the box to view the heart. Inside, there was a white, round, tall plastic container. Inside that container, my heart. We all wore plastic gloves; we put newspaper down on the table in case the liquid the heart was preserved in dripped. I removed my heart and held it in two hands because it was large, pale yellow, and deformed, but it hardly dripped. We passed it around and said thanks. Thanks to my old heart for doing all it could, thanks to the new heart for being so good, thanks to each other for coming home. I thought about the donor's family. It overwhelmed me to think that somewhere not so far away, there was someone young like me, small like me, with O-positive blood like mine, missing from a table. My family's gratitude, our joy, comes in large part from another family's grief. It's not a direct correlation, nor a direct result. I did not cause that death, but I did wait for it to come for a long time, and when it did, I was grateful. But what would that make the condition of my transplanted heart—not quite grieving, not quite gratitude? What can I call the crawl space in between?

The heart is called a "gift" from the donor to the recipient. I wonder if it's the right word for receiving, because you aren't just given a heart, you have to earn it. In the year I received a heart, only 2,167 heart transplants were performed off a list of over 4,000 waiting names. So there are levels of need, statuses of waiting that mark your closeness to death. Status 2 means you are in heart failure but not dying, because one can live in heart failure, just not very well. I lived in heart failure for seven years and it's difficult for me to say that any of them were bad, because I was a happy kid even though I did not know what wellness felt like. You are unlikely to receive a heart as a Status 2. Mostly, you bank time for when you become sicker and are bumped up to Status 1B or 1A. Status 1B means you are very sick, but you can live outside the hospital. Status 1A means you are at the end; you are holding death's hand. In theory, I suppose the levels make sense, but the complication comes because you can choose to make yourself sicker in order to bump yourself up on the list. Bumping up is common practice, a strategy, because if you wait too long, your other organs will start to fail. And if that happens, recovery after the transplant is more difficult and sometimes unsuccessful. The whole process feels like an exercise in how close you can get to death—close enough to earn a heart, not so close that the heart can't bring you back. There are other factors that also help or hinder receiving hearts—age, blood type (O blood will wait longer than most because anyone can receive an O, but only Os can save Os). I don't know all of them. I have always been too afraid to ask. Did it matter, for instance, that my family could afford good insurance, the surgery, and the drugs I'll always require? I'm not sure, but given the way health care functions in this country, I am inclined to think yes.

When you list as a child, before the age of eighteen as I did, you're also required to go through a psychological evaluation. Sometimes, kids lose themselves in their transplants and donors. They miss their illness because it made them special. Sometimes, donors can become a way of avoiding the overwhelming possibilities and responsibilities that come with wellness. Kids say they are living the life their donor left behind. I've struggled with what my obligations are to the donor, as well. It's a kind of self-preservation, I think, that I have not yet asked to know who the donor was. I might someday, but lately I think more about the space of grief in the transplant process. If it's possible to inhabit grief and gratitude at the same time, to respect the heart, the gift of it, and also believe it can never be truly earned or deserved.

In the Talmud, it says that Shimon bar Yochai, the paradigm for Jewish mystical teachers and miracle workers, lived with "one eye laughing and one eye crying." On the ten-year anniversary of the transplant, I go walking in the cemetery near my home in Iowa City. I make my way to the bodies-donated-to-science garden. There's a podium but nowhere to sit. I stand with an open notebook, ready to speak. I go up and down, up and down, on the balls of my feet. I don't pray often, and when pressed, I forget the words. Up down, up down. My father used to say that this motion, davening, is how angels pray—standing on their toes because their souls/soles are hot with holiness. But it's October and I'm cold standing in mist so fine that I can only see it when it lands on the pages of my open notebook. I press a hand to my chest; I search through my coat, the layers of shirts, for the heartbeat. How does it begin? I can't remember, so I walk in circles until my cheeks flush and I feel ready to take Death's hand. I whisper that I have been well, and then all the ways I am worried my life won't go right, all the ways I have embraced wellness: I might not be able to write a book; I might never find a partner; I might never have children; I might never get a haircut I like. Death kisses me slow, familiar, and I go quiet. I remember all the things I could not do before and, suddenly, the movement of my legs, the hunger in my stomach, the cold October morning, and my ability to stay warm are enough. We walk on and I recite the Mourner's Kaddish for the donor and the family for whom, ten years ago, they lost some light. I sit beside Death all morning, tracing the scar that runs up and down my chest. Ten years went so quickly, I say. I think of that picture my mother has in her phone of the cooler containing the heart. She told me she keeps it just to remember the moment. Maybe that's what the crawl space is between grief and gratitude—remembrance or memory. Maybe that is the condition of my transplanted heart, one of remembering.

Men Who Love
Dying Women and Fishing

Y OU NOTICE THE MAN BEFORE he speaks to you—late forties, graying hair around his temples, eager, wandering eyes hoping to make contact with someone, anyone, who might listen. You see him, not out of the corner of your eye but because of this sense you've developed as a small woman moving about the world. You notice, glancing up occasionally from your book, that he's moved tables a few times, quietly leaping closer to where you've been sitting for a few hours. Sometimes you think you read slower than most because you are always glancing up like a prairie dog, ready to run for your life. He's made it over to the table closest to you and is staring, waiting for your upward glance because you seem like the type of woman who will listen. And you are.

"It's almost my birthday," he says. "Just three weeks away."

Three weeks seems like a long time; three weeks doesn't seem like almost. You smile and wish him a happy early birthday. You keep your book open; you glance back down; you have no idea which paragraph you were reading. If only you were a faster, stronger mammal, you think.

"My wife's birthday is one week after mine," he says. "Happy early birthday to her, too. She died twelve years ago of heart failure."

You put your book down in your lap, closed but for one finger on the page you haven't finished reading. Twelve years ago you were eighteen, in heart failure, waiting for a transplant. For a moment, you think maybe this man can tell. You make eye contact; he leans forward.

"I'm sorry," you say.

Then he starts telling you about his dead wife.

"Our first date was at Red Lobster. We went somewhere else for dessert. After, she turned to me in the car and said she didn't want to go back to the nursing home, she wanted to come home and live with me."

"The nursing home?"

"Yeah, she was nine years my senior—forty-one. And sick. Heart failure. She told me all about it at the Red Lobster and I thought, Geez, y'know, just my luck—fall in love with a dying woman. But she was up front about it, gave me every opportunity to leave. She was dying, y'know?"

You nod. You do know dying; you do know heart failure. You know it makes you tired, so tired you can't make it up a flight of stairs on your own. You know it means that your heart is not able to pump the amount of blood necessary and at the right pace to make you hungry. You know eating becomes a task, something you must do even when you are nauseous. You know it's difficult to stay warm; you know the body doesn't pump enough blood to keep itself warm. You know you spent a lot of time in layers with blue lips, shivering. You know, but you don't tell the man how well. You don't tell him you also fell in love during heart failure. That you also gave that

67

man every opportunity to leave because you wondered, obsessively, over whether it was fair to ask someone to fall in love with a body that might not last. You wonder still, but now—ten years after the surgery and not in love—you also wonder whether you lost that first love to your wellness. Is there something to men loving dying women?

"She died right over there." He points out the window to a hospital down the street. "Well, no. Really she died in the ambulance on the way there. I watched her. I watched my wife die. That was hard. When we got to the hospital, they unloaded her and took her inside, but—" He shakes his head. "I called my buddy, the sheriff over in Johnson County." He asks if you know him, the sheriff. You do not. You've never committed a crime in Johnson County. "He came right away, middle of the night, all dressed in his sheriff's uniform, and sat with me. Sat with me until all the paperwork was done. He's a good buddy. He's my buddy. We go fishing every month. Last month we went and he caught a huge [name of a fish you don't know]."

Once, after the transplant, a man asking for money outside a café late at night called you Persephone, queen of the underworld. It was the only all-night café you knew of in St. Louis, and they allowed smoking inside and out. You were sitting with a new friend, sharing a cigarette. You both secretly loved cigarettes and staying up all night. You gave the man all the money you had, just a few bucks. He bowed to you, circled his heart with a long, pointed finger, took your hand in his, and kissed your palm.

"Thank you, my queen," he said, and then danced his way, trench coat dragging across cobblestones, to the next table.

Your friend laughed and suggested you go wash your hands. You walked inside to the bathroom and held your hand up to the fluorescent lights. You looked closely at your palm to see if maybe the man had left something there, some mark. His fingernails had been long, he'd traced them over your palm in circles the way he had over his heart, and his kiss was wet. You could've pulled away; he wasn't holding on so much as letting you rest there, your hand on his. You looked and looked at your palm, hoping something from his spit might remain. Something visible on your hand, something revelatory about living with this intimacy with death, something about Persephone living half her life in good company with death. But there was nothing but your palm and the light, bad love poems written in Sharpie on the bathroom wall, and dirty needles on the floor.

You looked in the mirror a long time to see if maybe something had revealed you to the man—if maybe your scars were showing or if you were once again pale, the way you used to be. You were still shocked at how pink your complexion was with all that good blood in you. You looked long enough to convince yourself that you could see the heart beating through your shirt. You walked out, bought a hot cup of coffee and a blueberry muffin that you intended to give to the man when you asked him what he meant when he called you Persephone. But by the time you stepped back outside, he was gone. Your friend told you the cops had come. You went back inside and asked the gawky young white man behind the counter, wearing a beanie on a warm night, if he had made the call to the police. He smiled at you and said yes, he had.

"Sorry I didn't do it sooner," he said. "Sorry you got kissed."

"Next time," you said, "you should ask."

He dropped his smile and said he hadn't made the call just for you; there were other customers he was bothering. You went back to sit with your friend, and she told you he went quietly, he seemed to know the officers, and it was a friendly exchange between them. You believed her, but isn't this always what people say when witnessing the removal of disorderly bodies—especially black bodies—that it's for their own good? Persephone, he said, a queen. You wonder if he could see something of your displaced heart in you, something of the secrecy in your body. You can't imagine how, because you've only ever been the kind of body that is seen as a beautiful, dying woman—delicate, hungry, and pale-skinned. You ate the muffin with your hands. You licked your fingers, and it was only then that you remembered you never washed your palm.

The fishing story continues, and you start to think that the metaphor here is that waiting for fish is like listening to this story about waiting for fish. You're starting to plan your exit from this man made unstable by grief but also probably by something that happened to him before grief. What was it before grief that made him love a dying woman? A woman who couldn't get hungry, couldn't take long walks. A woman who was pale and thin, a woman who wouldn't last.

When you see pictures of yourself from heart failure, you think you look too young. You wanted pictures just before the surgery to remember your before body because everything would change. Your sister took Polaroids of you in the shower just before you went to the hospital. Photos of your chest and face, your thin arms. You wanted the memory of your body, the body people called "waiflike" and "lithe." The chest that would soon be cut, broken, and stapled together again. And when you look at the photos, you sometimes think what a tender time heart failure was. You were dying, sure, but because of dying, every-thing, everything, was a gift. And you weren't hungry or worried about what you wanted, only what you could have. There were times you didn't mind dying because it kept you so full.

"What was your wife's name?" you ask, inter-rupting the time the sheriff from Johnson caught another fish whose name you do not know.

The man tells you her name and it's a name that always sounds young. It's a name that belongs to girls in pigtails wearing floral jumpers.

"She was forty-one when she died," he says. "I'm forty-five now. My brother says I should date, and I have, but—I don't like pushy women. I tried. I dated a woman. But she wanted so much from me, wanted me to do things and change. I didn't like that. I dropped her."

You don't tell the man about your heart. Forty-one is not old and you don't know why she died; you don't know why you didn't. But also, you think, he's not looking to really talk with you. He hasn't even asked you your name.

"I don't date women with records. If you've committed a crime, messed around with drugs, I don't want you. I don't date women who drink or smoke or talk too much. If I can't get a word in, I don't want you. I don't date fat women. I keep in shape, so you should, too. I don't date women who insist on paying for—"

"What made you stay with your wife?" you say.

"What?"

"When you found out she was in heart failure, what made you stay?"

"Oh. I guess you're right. I gave her a second chance, maybe I should give women with records one, too."

You didn't mean that, but okay, sure. "What made you stay?"

She was beautiful. He describes her and she doesn't look like you. You are relieved.

"And I loved her, what could I do? We were married two years and three months."

You think of Frank Sinatra singing: . . . *sue me / Sue me / What can you do me / I love you.*

"We played pranks, my wife and me. She put a mousetrap in my shoe once."

Give a holler and hate me / Hate me / Go ahead, hate me! / I love you.

"I put tacks on the toilet seat. She whacked me in the head when I got home from work. I had a concussion!"

Sue me, sue me. / Shoot bullets through me / I love you!

"Do you like pranks?" he asks.

"No, not really."

He tells you his name and you offer yours.

"Athena?" he says.

"Adina."

"Atweena?"

"Adina—with a *d*, like a dog."

"Tina?"

"Yes. Tina."

"You're real nice, Tina. Not a lot of nice women left."

"Thank you. I have to go now. I have dinner plans. It was nice meeting you."

"You, too, Tina."

You get up to leave and he reaches his hand out. You take it.

"You know what my wife hated the most? When I would tickle her ribs. Women hate that, when you tickle their ribs and won't stop. I bet you would hate that, Tina. If someone tickled your ribs?"

He's still holding your hand and you know this was all avoidable had you just said, I'm sorry for your loss, and left over an hour ago.

"Yes, I would hate it. And it wouldn't be funny, I would just hate it."

"Okay, Tina. I can tell you mean business. You're nice, though."

"I'll see you around." You take back your hand.

"Yeah. Be seeing you, Tina."

You walk outside and think about how awful being tickled by a stranger in public would have been. You kick yourself for losing an hour of your life to someone who hates fat women and women with criminal records. You call yourself Tina in your mind as a punishment. Dumb Tina, why did you stay? Why do you care so much to know why the man in the coffee shop fell in love with a woman who died? Why did you stay?

I don't know. Something about loving dying women and fishing, I guess.

Your Heart, Your Scars, Zombies

A WEEK OR SO AFTER MY twenty-first birth-day, a little over a year after the heart transplant I received at age nineteen, K picked me up outside my dorm and we drove to Blueberry Hill for my first legal beer. I'd had the stomach flu and finals on my actual birthday, so I hadn't done much celebrating yet. He ordered for me, a Blue Moon with an orange slice. I didn't tell him I preferred darker beers. We sat across from each other in a booth. I don't remember what we talked about, but I do remember the talking was easy and I liked his smile.

We'd been out on other dates, but we were not dating. We'd gone and listened to live music at local bars, we'd slow-danced late at night at house parties, but I was still in love with a boyfriend from high school who went off to college while I stayed home in St. Louis to wait for a heart. The boyfriend and I had been together a long time by college standards. We were each other's dates for senior prom, and he flew home from college when the heart came. While I was in surgery, he made me a list of all the things he knew about me— what I loved and hated, how I picked out onions and scallions from soup, where I liked to be kissed—so that I would have it to refer to when I woke up with a dead person's heart in place of my own. The items on the list were things to remember, what made me Adina to him, just in case that foreign heart should cause me to forget. We lived together over the summer after the surgery and decided that seeing other people in our junior year was best because we both wanted to study abroad but at different times. K understood all this—he and his high school girlfriend had been through the same standard study-abroad breakup. I hadn't mentioned the heart transplant part of the story, though. Maybe because it was so nice when K would say, "Yes, I went through exactly the same thing." When he would ask if we could kiss, I'd say I wasn't ready to break the boyfriend's heart in exactly that way just yet. This was true, but I had also never been naked with someone who didn't know the history of my body, the origin of my scars, and maybe I wasn't quite ready for that, either. So when he drove me back to my dorm, on the cusp of winter break, and we sat there watching our still-visible breath in the cold of his car, I hoped he wouldn't ask again.

"I made you something," he said. He pulled a case out of his pocket and popped a CD he had burned from his laptop into his portable car stereo, the nicest part of his old SUV. The songs were all by K, written and performed. Mostly they were honky-tonk-like country songs, along with a slow acoustic cover of Miley Cyrus's "Party in the USA." As the first song played, I realized it was about me.

No one had ever written me songs before, and I wasn't sure how I was supposed to listen to them. Should I meet his eyes as lyrics about taking down my tall other man and longing for me hit the air? I chose to stare at the stereo instead and sort of smile. I said something about being impressed that he had the time to make the CD between working on his thesis, finals, and applying for a Fulbright. This was maybe not the response he was hoping for. He asked if my roommates were all gone for winter break already. They were. Could we listen to the rest of the CD inside my dorm? It was getting late, past eleven, and the boyfriend had texted me that his flight had landed, he was home, a ten-minute drive away, and would love to see me.

"I'm sorry, K, but I'm still not ready for that," I said.

He lowered the volume on the stereo. "I don't know if it helps," he said, "but your friends told me about you." He looked down at his hands. "They told me about your heart."

He went on to say that he liked scars and horror movies. He had scars himself from a trauma, and he liked the aesthetics of horror. He loved, he said, the aesthetics of zombie movies. He was excited to see my body. He was sure, in this way, he would find it beautiful. Heat filled the car as

81

he talked, and I could no longer see my breath. I don't remember where I put my eyes while he talked—maybe out the windshield at the deserted campus, maybe on the stereo still playing songs about brown hair, brown eyes, mine.

Your heart . . .

Your scar . . .

Zombie movies.

♥

IT IS INCREDIBLE TO BE ABLE to live with a dead person's heart. Not only live but thrive. It's almost unthinkable. Prior to the transplant, I asked countless questions of anyone who would sit with me about the implications of living with a dead person's heart. Who would I be when I woke up? Who would I love? What would I remember? The boyfriend's solution was the list—to hand me back to myself when I woke up from that deep, cutting sleep.

I, on the other hand, read articles on cellular memory, the theory that our cells—blood, organs, etc.—house memories in our body. I read articles, reputable and not, that claimed sometimes organ recipients wake up with memories that aren't theirs, with love for people they've never met, with feelings they cannot locate within their own histories. The most memorable of these stories was about a young boy who received a heart from another young boy and upon being in a room with the donor's mother, having no knowledge of who she was or what she looked like, the recipient ran to the woman and hugged her legs in the way that small children do with mothers. When asked why, the boy replied that he loved her. I wondered then what got in and what would be taken out. I worried then that I might not recognize my mother by heart when I awoke, as I had before. I had not considered zombies.

The modern Western appropriation of the zombie is often read as a metaphor for pure capitalism. George Romero's zombie films of the 1970s and '80s, like *Dawn of the Dead* and *Day of the Dead*, ushered in the flesh-eating, blind consumer element to the monster. Prior to these films, the zombie body served a different purpose. The myth of the zombie originates in Haiti. A dead body—one that is in a state of unrest from either improper burial or improper death—is raised by someone who then becomes the zombie master. In this narrative, the zombie body is nonviolent, nonfeeling, and nonconsuming. Most often, raised zombies are used to work the fields. In this way, the zombie of Haitian origins becomes an allegory for slavery, for the body of the Other, and for an emptiness that allows the creator to inscribe meaning and impose work.

The zombie can also be read as a body that challenges the binary of life and death, creating a third, some have argued queer, space between living and not living. Marc Leverette, zombie scholar, refers to this category as a "corpse that is no longer an I" or "Thanatos in drag." Thanatos, in Greek mythology, is a demonic representation of death. He rarely appears in myths and is not the same as Hades, god of death. Thanatos does not control death but is death. In one myth, Thanatos is ordered by Zeus to chain Sisyphus to the underworld because it is time for him to die. Sisyphus, however, manages to overcome Thanatos and instead chains the god to his own restraints. While Thanatos is chained, no one on Earth can die. Thanatos is eventually freed and death continues. A zombie, therefore, is death walking around the world looking like life.

The change from heart failure to wellness had been quick, and most days after the transplant, I did walk about the world feeling a lot like death in drag. I had gone from not being able to walk half a mile without resting to thinking I'd like to travel to study clowning in Italy in less than one year. I needed only to walk to and from classes, spend all day out of bed, or dance at night at a party to feel amazement and gratitude for this different heart. Inside of that gratitude was the realization that I might never feel as if being healthy and having energy is normal. I might never really belong among my peers, the healthy. Once in an acting class, someone told me I was exciting to watch because I had instincts and made choices in scenes that no human really did but it worked and it was funny. In other words, I was weird.

I woke up one morning a few months after the surgery exhausted, unable to get out of bed. I called my mother in terror, crying uncontrollably that it was all over, the transplant had failed, and I was once again dying. I think you have a cold, she said. I think you're regular-people sick. We laughed for the same reason I was funny in acting class—what did I know about regular people, what did I know about healthy? I was still learning how to inhabit this strange third space between death and life. Dependent on death and reanimated body parts, oddly grateful for the gift death allowed, and now undeniably alive but marked with difference. So when K turned to me when we first met, before zombies and hearts, and said, "I understand your heartbreak, I went through the same thing," I felt, maybe, what it was to belong. To be regular-people broken, to be heartsick over lost love and nothing more.

Donors and recipients both are bodies inhabiting a third space of living and not living. Hearts don't come from corpses, but a more specific kind of death—brain death. When organs from "dead" donors are harvested, the heart continues to beat until it is the last piece of the body to be cut out. It then ceases to be living, ceases to function. It is put on ice, in a cooler, and transported to the recipient's body, where it is reattached, revived, reanimated, bringing both heart and recipient back to life. In my imagination that morning I woke with a cold, some amorphous being came to me, demanding back the heart. It wasn't the donor, necessarily, but whatever it was, was perhaps zombielike. A corpse without a heart, a stumbling, empty person reaching out for lost life. And somehow, in my imagining, should the zombie find me, reclaim the heart, it would not leave me dead, but back where I started, because in my childhood bedroom, in a box on my nightstand, preserved in some scentless chemical, sits my old heart. I kept it. It's not normal to keep old hearts; it's not standard. But I insisted, and when asked why by doctors who thought it strange, I replied, "Because it is mine."

To be clear, I don't think of putting my heart back in my chest; that's not the reason for keeping it. On a simple level, it served me for nineteen years and I couldn't bear to think of it thrown away as medical waste after a biopsy. Call me a romantic. But I also had all those questions: What lived there? What was taken out? What lies sleeping in a dying heart? The questions are unanswerable, but the heart's presence gives me comfort perhaps simply because it is undeniably mine. It has never belonged to anyone else. It is perhaps the only thing now outside my body that will ever be truly mine. Is it greedy to have two hearts, one living and one dead? Possibly. Is it a kind of horror? Probably. Is it zombielike? No, not really.

The zombie body is one without purpose, without desire, empty. It is this emptiness, this new relation to death, this body of difference that is neither alive nor buried that offers opportunity to discuss what about this radical, nonbinary body terrifies or enthralls. What can be written on a blank body of difference? How can it be read or interpreted? Perhaps if you can name another's alterity, you can maybe control that body, make it work for you, make it useful. For a slave narrative, it can be said that the body was created to work, focusing on its usefulness and not its humanity. What, then, for an illness narrative? Perhaps that I am what you make me—I live in this way, a different body, a body of hybridity, to mean something to you, to your experiences, to practice your empathy, to fetishize, even to "inspire." But perhaps keeping my heart complicates this. Perhaps the horror of keeping a useless heart in a box on one's nightstand can be read as a feminist act: at once a declaration of ownership and a way of denying possession or being possessed. A part of the body horrifically claimed. I am not empty but twofold, abundant.

♥

BACK IN THE CAR WITH K, the reanimated heart pounding in my chest, my little zombie, I could not find the courage to ask him: K, am I, then, your zombie?

89

No, of course not. And I'm sure K would agree. He did not mean to other me; he did not mean to give name to my difference. He meant, I think, to woo me. With songs, with understanding, with excitement for my specific body. I regret that when he stopped talking, I didn't ask what he meant by linking my heart, my scars, and my nakedness to the undead. I was twenty-one; no one had ever written me songs before or called me a zombie. I didn't know how to have a conversation about what it might mean.

Instead, after he stopped talking, there was a long pause between us. Finally, I said, "It's not really like that. It's a clean scar, not zombielike. You might be disappointed." He laughed and assured me he would find everything surrounding my scar exciting, as well. I repeated that I wasn't ready. I thanked him for the CD of songs about longing and said it was time for me to go inside. He gave me the CD, hugged me outside the car, and asked once more if he could kiss me.

"No," I said without guilt or apology.

When he drove away, I allowed myself to cry. Your heart, your scars, zombies. You do not belong here—you are not fully, or maybe too fully, alive. I went inside my dorm, took off all my clothes in the hallway, and showered. I texted "Come over" to the boyfriend and redressed.

When he arrived, I didn't mention K or zombies. It was nearly midnight, but the awkwardness of being unsure where we stood with each other, if either of us had slept with someone else, drove us to sit on my couch, untouching, and watch a movie rather than talk. My roommates had ordered *La Vie en Rose* from Netflix, and neither of us had seen it. I turned off all the lights, and during the opening scene, as Edith Piaf began to sing, I climbed on top of him and took off my shirt. He laughed. "Oh, thank God," he said. "I thought we were going to watch this whole movie." We kissed, and when he whispered how much he had missed me, he called me nothing but by my name.

Should You Hold Me Down
(Go on, Take It)

"WILL I FEEL IT?" I ASK THE DOCTOR as I do a slight hop onto the operating table. He turns to me while pulling on his gloves. "Latex allergy," I say, lifting my wrist to show him my plastic bracelet that says just that.

"What happens when you come into contact with latex?"

My eyes meet the resident's gaze and he quickly looks away, blushing. He's about my age, I guess, and suddenly I'm conscious of the sheerness of my hospital gown and the outline of my breasts. If he looks closely enough, he might be able to see my new heart pounding, my chest rising and falling from the beat, my skin pulled tight like a drum over the new instrument. I think about telling the doctor the truth: If I take it in my mouth, nothing happens, but if I have sex with latex condoms, it burns for days. Instead, I look at the floor and say, "Rash."

The doctor switches his gloves and tells me to "lay down." It's *lie*, I think.

Instruments start moving, metal-on-metal sounds, and I whip my head from one direction to another, trying to see. The nurse pulls my hair back into a shower cap and tells me that I'm so pretty, she didn't think I was a patient when she came out to call my name in the waiting room. I smile at her and resist the urge to ask what other patients look like. She means it as a kindness, I know. But *pretty* is the wrong word, I want to tell her. The truth is, we don't really have a word to describe a woman who comes through something a lot like death and remains light. We don't have it for boys, either, so we say *strong* for them. We say *pretty* when we mean *you look a lot like life.*

I thank her and ask, "Do you strap me in? Should you hold me down?"

93

"Haven't you had a lot of these?" the doctor asks.

"I was always asleep."

"Why?"

"Because I was a kid, I guess. Because I might try to run, maybe." I smile at my small attempt at a joke. I smile and make jokes in these situations because I think that people, doctors, are more likely to want to keep funny people alive. The doctor laughs as he holds up the catheter, the small needle he plans to insert into the base of my neck, and then cast a thin line down into my heart. The nurse stands to my right and strokes my hair. I take a deep breath to slow my heart and I think about how biopsies used to be for me when I was younger. The walls of the lab at St. Louis Children's Hospital were painted with stars. Maybe because it was comforting to think of something like this happening in the dead of night, when a kid could sleep through it, wake up six hours later still a little drugged, saying, And you were there, and you, and you. But inevitably, that kid would reach her hand up to the sore spot at the base of her neck and realize it had all been real, in some way, those minutes when someone was taking pieces of her heart.

Here, in this new hospital, the nurse tells me that during the procedure I should pick a spot on the wall to focus on. I search the wall for stars, but there are only patches of more white and less white. I choose less, just above my head.

The nurse tells me that she's going to insert the IV now. "Better you don't look, sweetheart," she says.

"I'm a really difficult stick," I say. "But this vein, *this* vein is good." I point to a spot in the crook of my arm, to the veins that have held IVs successfully in the past and still retain just the faintest mark of tiny blue dots. I want to ask the nurse to count to three, to make sure I'm ready so that I can breathe deeply to try to stay relaxed to prevent the vein from contracting, and to please not dig, because, truly, it's not the sticks that I mind; it's only the digging around, the rooting for the vein in my skin, that sometimes makes me cry, because I had this nurse once and she shoved a needle in my arm and she wouldn't pull it out even after I screamed *Stop.* I want to give her that speech, the speech I always give nurses before IVs, but they don't count to three here and I feel silly asking. I just point to the crook of my right arm.

"That's the best spot," I say. "And, if it's okay, can I have a twenty-four needle?"

"That's too small," the doctor says.

"I know it's for babies," I say. "But anything bigger usually blows the vein."

"I'd like to try a twenty first," the doctor says.

"I'm sorry," I say, "but I'd really prefer the twenty-four. You're not giving me much, right? I'm going to be awake the whole time, right?"

The nurse laughs. "Wow, somebody's an expert. I think a twenty-four is fine. I pulled one anyway when I saw how tiny you are."

"Thank you," I say.

"Are you ready, sweetheart?" she asks. I nod and the IV is inserted. I want to close my eyes, but I don't because I'm not sure if that might be rude, and I feel like I've gained some clout with the needle talk. Once it's in, I thank the nurse and tell her it wasn't so bad.

The doctor tells me that first he'll numb my neck using a shot. "It might burn," he says.

The nurse holds my head firmly to the right and says, "Got your point?"

I smile and say yes, though, really, I can't find one and all I can think is, *Why did I need an IV if you're going to give me a shot in my neck and no drugs to put me to sleep?*

The shot burns and I try to concentrate on not moving, not looking around, not thinking about the size of the needle in my neck. I focus on my breathing and think that maybe this counts as going to yoga.

"I'm going to start now," the doctor says, "threading the catheter to your heart. You might feel it skip a few beats. You might feel it, y'know, react. Inhale deep and hold it."

I inhale. I close my eyes.

♥

SUMMER. THE WINDOWS ARE OPEN in the attic, where our friends decide to re-create their childhood game of turning off the lights and running around the room, leaping over furniture, and avoiding whoever is "it." I guess it's tag, just in the dark, and slightly more erotic because you seem to grab at one another, tackle one another to the ground, and then cry out when you've lost. But we're older now and drunk, and I'd rather be out driving with you on our favorite streets with the windows down and the smells of honeysuckle, humidity, and sweat filling the space between us. Instead, we're in this attic, trapped with other people. The sky is clear, and light from the stars comes in through the window, so that it's not quite pitch-black. I'm by the open window, just sitting because I think this game is sort of dumb. But then you find me under the window, in the dark. You grab my ankle, wrapping your whole hand around its smallness. You drag my body down beneath yours on the carpet and I reach up to find your curls, to make sure it's you. I know you by the way you take my fingers in your mouth when I reach up to find your face. I laugh and turn my neck to the right. I cover my mouth to stay quiet. You start to kiss a line down my neck to my clavicle. I imagine you're drawing a clear path to my heart with the wetness of your kisses. Someone cries out that they've been found, and you move across the room in three strides as the lights come on. I can feel your spit drying on my skin and a faint pulse at the base of my neck from where you lingered before the lights came on. *Let's play again*, I say. You look down at the dirty shag carpet and blush, your cheeks turning a pink I've never found so pretty.

♥

"I'M IN NOW," THE DOCTOR SAYS.

"Okay?" the nurse asks.

"I thought it would be more painful," I say.

"Nah. I'll take a few pieces. You'll feel a tug, though, when they come out," the doctor says.

The nurse asks if I'm comfortable, because she's noticed that my cheeks are warm and flushed.

"Yes," I say, "it's just different."

"Think of something else, sweetheart," she says.

♥

IN THE EMPTY BEDROOM in your basement, I watch you remove each piece of your mother's clothing drying atop towels on the unmade twin bed. I mock you as you fold the clothes meticulously because you think that one tank top out of place, one wrinkled pair of Jockeys, and she might know that we had sex. When you finish, you sit on the bed. I close the door and the windowless room is pitch-black. I open it again, just a crack, so the light can get in. You hold out your hands and pull me to your chest.

We've already been up all night kissing, and usually it stops there, on the couch, but I want to have sex at least once with you before the transplant. My eyelids are heavy and my lips are chapped. We take off each other's clothes with surprising ease. We lie down together, and with my arm draped across your chest and my head in the crook of your shoulder, I understand how this works so well: your bigness and my smallness, how we fit like a puzzle.

You prop yourself on top of me. You kiss my eyelids. *Don't fall asleep, don't fall asleep,* you say. You continue to kiss your way down my neck to my breasts and finally to the jagged scar in the center of my chest. You trace the scar with your fingers. I like to think that your touch, your saliva, takes it all away, this boundary between my left and right breast. This part of myself I spend away from you in the hospital. You trace the line with your tongue, soft at first and then almost lapping, as if you really could lick it clean. I curl my fingers in your hair and tell you how I used to dream that a man would kiss my scars and how I never imagined licking would be better. You laugh and say, *I'll lick the new one, too.*

♥

THE NURSE STROKES MY HAIR. "Are you having any pain?" she asks.

"No," I say, "not pain, exactly."

"Can you feel it?" the nurse asks.

"Yes. When the pieces come out," I say. "There's a tug. It's incredible."

"I'll need six or seven pieces," the doctor says. "For accuracy."

The nurse reminds me to breathe.

♥

ON THE THANKSGIVING FOLLOWING the transplant, after the turkey, after everyone goes around the table and says they're grateful I'm still there, after the guests leave, I call you and ask if you'd like to come see my heart. When you arrive, I kiss you on the stoop. You swipe your thumb over my cheek. *Pink*, you say. I guide you inside to the kitchen. The rest of my family sits around the table, the wooden box in the center, a screwdriver beside it. My mother has covered the table in old newspapers, as if we've all gathered to decoupage. You give quick hugs to everyone and sit in the one empty chair. I start unscrewing the bottom of the box. One of the screws sticks and my brother asks if I want help. He finishes the rest and the bottom comes off. Inside, there's a plastic container not unlike what soup from a take-out restaurant might come in. My mother tells me to wait, that we all need gloves if we're going to touch it. The nonlatex gloves appear on the table very quickly. The gloves are big on my hands, small on yours. Everyone holds their hands just above the table, as if they all need to stay sterile, as if the surgery has yet to come. I pop the top of the container and, to my surprise, there's no smell. I smile and say, *It's in pieces.* My mother explains that they biopsied it first. They sliced my heart up. Everyone nods as if yes, of course, of course they would slice it up. I pick up the biggest piece with my right hand, and it's bigger than my fist. Maybe even bigger than yours. And it's yellow, like the yolk of a hard-boiled egg, and pieces of what look like wet tissue paper coat the unclean thing. I wonder why it's yellow, if it's maybe from being exposed to the air, or if it was that color inside of me. My mother reminds me that the doctors had said it was done working, and I was lucky it came out when it did. *That's the color of a dead heart*, she says. I pass the heart around the table, and when it comes to you, you set it on your palm and bend your neck to see inside.

♥

"WHEN YOU TAKE THE PIECES," I ask the doctor, "do they grow back?"

The silent resident furrows his brow and looks to the doctor as if, maybe, he's just not sure.

"No," the doctor answers to the whole room. "They don't grow back."

"Oh," I say. "Just wondering."

♥

YOU CALL ME ONE NIGHT, walking around your cold mountain college town, and ask if we can talk. You tell me that you miss me every day but that you're feeling lost and it's me, maybe, how I've always been beautiful and you're only now realizing your own curly hair, your own strength, your own perfect hands. You say, *Maybe we should see other people.* You say, *I just want to be sure.* You tell me that you don't want to call each other mine anymore but that if anyone else ever did, you would die. You say, *I would die* lightly, as if I didn't come so close, as if it was more than just six months ago that you sat on the edge of your college XL bed, searching for a plane ticket home at any cost while I lay in surgery. I can hear it in your voice: You're the least likely to go and the most likely to be left behind. We hang up and a moment later my phone vibrates with your text. *Please don't forget to take your pills.*

♥

"Don't worry," the doctor says. "This heart is plenty big. Looks healthy, too. How old is it?"

"I guess it's six years old," I say. "Or, rather, I've had it for six years."

"Still young," the doctor says.

He tells me to take a big breath and hold it as he pulls the catheter away from my heart,

105

through my chest, up out of my neck. I assume it's safe to exhale now, but no one has told me so, and the feeling of the catheter coming out of my neck has left me breathless. The nurse is ready with gauze and presses firmly on the entry site.

♥

END OF SUMMER. OUTSIDE OF MY HOUSE, we sit in the car, listening to the radio. I notice that your smell has changed. It's been good, this time away from each other. I've been traveling. I've been happy. I think about the times I was too sick to walk up the stairs and you carried me to bed. When we were grateful just for my health. I ask how your summer was; I ask about our friends. You tell me that your summer was fine and that maybe we've outgrown each other. You tell me that maybe I'm just not the kind of woman you'd ever want to marry. That you hope we can still be friends. I think about all the times you've held me in this car with the radio playing, all the times I needed you and you carried me. I put my hand on the door handle and warn you that I'm going, the way I used to do when we were first together and I wanted you to kiss me. I'm barely breathing but ask if you're okay. *I'm fine*, you say, *it's just not you.* I open the door of your car. I have nothing left to say because you're not really here. I give you one last chance to tell me that you still love me more than anything and that you'd like to lick me clean again or, rather, you'd like to try. But instead, you watch me walk inside my house, see my mother there ready to receive me with a hug, and, as you drive away, you call that girl from the summer. The girl who didn't make you feel that when she wasn't around, the world was fine and fun and lacking only her; the girl who didn't make you think of all that you lack.

♥

"WOULD YOU LIKE TO SEE THEM?" the doctor asks. "The little pieces of your heart?"

I'm surprised he asks. Maybe, like the nurse said, I'm so small and I must've been even smaller before the surgery (yes, I told her, eighty-six pounds), yet still such a pretty patient, and, somehow, that makes it—the scars, the flaws, the imperfections written on my body—all the more unfortunate.

I press the gauze to my neck to help the blood clot as the doctor hands me a small container with six floating pink flecks. He shakes it a bit, like a snow globe, so that the pieces of my heart flitter about in the liquid. *Ho, ho, ho, little girl*, I think.

"Wow," I say. "They're so pink." The doctor laughs and asks what color I thought they'd be.

"It's just that my old heart was yellow," I say.

A silence spreads through the room. I don't bother looking up to comfort them.

"How do you know that?" the doctor asks.

"I kept it," I say.

I turn the plastic over in my hands and remember the old heart, how it worked so hard to be enough, how it gave all it could, how I'd held it in my hands after it was out and had planned to thank it for all it had given me, but it was yellow and I resented it for not letting me know sooner that it was cooked.

"Pink," I say again, almost in a trance.

"If you laugh today," the nurse says, "keep pressure on your neck so that you don't bleed."

I thank the doctor, I hug the nurse, and I shake the resident's hand, all while holding on to the container.

"I'll need that back." The doctor laughs. "Unless you plan on keeping everything that comes out of your body."

I give the little container one last shake and watch the pieces float to the bottom as I hand it to the doctor. The nurse starts to escort me back to the waiting area. I remind myself: *This heart is plenty big.*

"Did you feel the tug?" the doctor asks as I walk out the door.

"Yeah," I say.

"Did it make you feel good?"

Thank God for the Nights
That Go Right

I STOOD NEXT TO A MAN at a bar with a four-dollar beer in one hand, my coat in the other, and no good way to grab my pills at 10:00 P.M. I'd spent a lot of nights at bars that week and I'd missed my 10:00 P.M. deadline more than once. It's the easiest thing, the only thing I have to do, really, to stay alive—just take the pills at the same time every morning and every night in order to have the perfect amount of medicine in my system so that my body doesn't suddenly wake up and say, *Fuck this heart, rip it up, it doesn't belong.* And still, sometimes, I forget, I slip up, I'm late. If 10:00 P.M. becomes 10:15 P.M., that's okay, that's not too bad. If 10:15 P.M. becomes 11:00 P.M., that's no good, that's missing the half-hour window I was once told I had. Then I take them with a swig of beer, a sip of whiskey, a shot of tequila once, and I think, *Well, look at you, you undeserving idiot.* But I've been lucky, we say, I've been so very lucky. Not one bit of rejection, not a one, sometimes in spite of me.

I didn't know much about the man. Or, rather, I knew a few small things and one large thing. We'd both had heart transplants. It's not really bar talk.

He was a friend of my friend Joey. Joey was the friend I called first when we knew the heart was coming, the friend who sat on my bed as I packed my bag for the hospital, the friend who got me through, the best friend. She was part of a house improv team at the Upright Citizen's Brigade with the man; they practiced and performed every week. I'd met him once before. I'd been helping Joey make papier-mâché piñatas for hours for an upcoming comedy show. When the man showed up, I was covered in homemade paste and a little wound up. Apparently, he thought I was funny and "super weird." Months later, Joey called me late one night when she was walking home from rehearsal, after he'd told her that he'd had a heart transplant. She talks fast when she's excited.

"I can't believe I didn't know," I said.

"How would you know?" she said. "You'd never know with you."

"I guess I just expected to be able to, like, smell it on someone else," I said.

"That's so crazy. Don't tell anyone you think that. He's fourteen years out," she said. "Fourteen."

Before the transplant, doctors told me a new heart would last for ten good years. Not just ten years but ten good years. After that, the kidneys might start to fail from one kind of immunosuppressant, you might get skin cancer from another, or the arteries might start to harden for reasons they can't quite explain. I was at seven and doing, as one doctor put it, beautifully—I'd had no rejection, no hardening of the arteries, no signs of decline in any other organ. There are reasons for all these things—better medicines, a good diet, etc.—but I am more comfortable calling it luck.

Still, the phrase "ten good years" lingers in my head and Joey knows it well.

"Fourteen?" I said. "Really?"

"Yeah," she said. "Fourteen. And he drinks *a lot*. Maybe you guys should get together, maybe that'd be nice."

"Yeah," I said. "I'd like to race him."

I went to their next improv show alone. After, I went down to the basement bathroom of the theater before meeting Joey at the adjacent bar. In the bathroom, I checked that I didn't have any eyeliner or mascara clumps in the corners of my eyes. I was nervous, like I was maybe about to go on what would be the worst blind date ever.

I found Joey at the bar. She asked if I wanted her to reintroduce me to the man with fourteen years, if I was sure. I thanked her for asking. It is nice to have a friend who holds my secrets like they are her secrets, too.

I shook his hand like we'd never met before, and one of the other members of the improv team standing nearby said, "Hey, you guys are heart twins!" Not really, I thought, because that's not a thing, thank God. We stepped over to the bar together to get drinks and talk about this largeness between us. I ordered a Porkslap.

We talked about what meds we were each on and what doctors we saw in the city. We'd seen the same cardiologist at one time, but he'd switched. He didn't get many checkups anymore—just an annual, almost like any other red-blooded American.

"Me, too, sort of," I said. I explained that I had gone to India recently, so they'd made me get every shot imaginable and then come by for a few checkups after the trip. I think we cheers'd to that.

The man was not tall. He had blue eyes and wholesome boy hair—soft, golden brown, buzzed. He looked like he was in his twenties but was, Joey said, at least thirty-two and just had nice skin. He wore his pink oxford shirt untucked from his khakis but buttoned to the top. Maybe, I thought, to cover his scar.

He'd had his transplant in Maryland during college. "Mine was during college, too," I said. "In St. Louis. Joey was there." He asked why I needed it. I told him I was in heart failure from the time I was twelve and that I had waited for the heart for nearly two years. His story was different. He'd never had any issues growing up, but he got sick in college, an infection or something, and needed a transplant immediately—he waited for less than two weeks. You're fast, I'm slow, I thought. Your trauma must be so different from mine. I imagined what it would be like to think of yourself as healthy all of your life and then be suddenly not. I couldn't, really, because I have never had that sort of training. It must have been terrifying. Before my transplant, I spoke on the phone once to a man who had had two heart transplants in his life. He grew up in the same town as my mother; they went on a date once. He said the only difference he notices is that his heart takes a little longer to catch up to him when he exercises, that there's a slight delay, and he can't work out quite as hard as he used to or ski from as high an altitude. "That won't be a problem for you," he'd said. "You have nothing to compare it to." He was right.

I wondered if the man in front of me was similar, if maybe the memory of wellness still lived in his body. There were long, awkward pauses during our conversation at the bar when I should've been asking him more questions—him at fourteen years, nice, and willing to answer. But I couldn't even make proper eye contact with him. The questions I still have— the ones about death and donors and borrowed time—seemed out of place standing at the bar, Porkslap in one hand and heart in the other. So I asked instead what he was up to now. He worked in health care. "To give back," he said.

I put my coat between my knees and checked the time on my phone: 10:35 P.M. I mentally kicked myself around for failing to check the clock earlier and dug in my bag for my medicine. I took it fast with a swig of beer and the man told me he took his pills at nine and nine. He said something about my looking good, something along the lines of being surprised when Joey told him I'd had a transplant. I didn't know what to say. I should; it's something I've heard a lot in the years since I received the heart. That I am un-patient-like; that you cannot tell, with my clothes on, the freakishness of my distinctly modern body. As if illness should be uglier, more grotesque. I should have said that I, too, was surprised by his wellness, his unfreakishness. I was afraid, however, that he might take it as flirting. There is no part of me that wants to be with someone who has scars like mine or scars at all. In bars, in life, I am drawn to men who are like trees—tall and strong, the opposite of myself. Men who have not spent time in hospitals, men whose bodies seem to be lottery winners, rare forms of perfection who make me feel, in the times we are together, that I belong in that club of plain and unsurprising beauty.

Joey came over. I'm not sure if it was by luck or because she noticed the man and I weren't really talking anymore. She said she had to run to another show. I told her I'd walk with her to the subway. I said good-bye and nice to re-meet you to Mr. Fourteen Years.

117

While we were walking to the train, I apologized to Joey. I told her I was weird and awkward with her friend.

"I kind of lost it when he said he worked in health care," I said.

"Why?" she asked.

"I don't know. He's just so *together*. He was probably like, *That girl is covered in trauma.*"

"I don't think people think like that," Joey said. "I'm sure it was weird for him, too. Are you okay?"

"I think so. I just feel shitty, like a shit person, a person made of shit."

She gave me a hug, patted me on my head like she sometimes does, and told me to give myself a break. We boarded the F train, going in opposite directions, and I thought about my seven years since the transplant. I'd graduated from college, moved to New York, worked at internships in theater and publishing, and done odd jobs—nannying, personal assistant, retail—until I'd landed at a literary magazine. Transplant aside,

I was like every other upper-middle-class white female riding this gentrification train back to Brooklyn. I was failing, I thought, being selfish with this new heart. I'd never struggled with failure before. When you're concentrated on survival, getting through, or making the best of things, you succeed by adapting. Failure only becomes a possibility when you have something to lose. With wellness, I suddenly had so much to waste. I could waste my time, my body, my heart on anything and I was starting to miss the strong muscle of gratitude I had built during my childhood through having to make hard choices about where I would spend what little energy I had.

After seven years, my gratitude is becoming less tangible. Some days I waste myself on bad television, on food that will clog arteries, on selfishness. And I tell myself it doesn't matter because even on that day, I am growing older and that is all I need do to deserve this "gift." I tell myself I will be grateful tomorrow. I am starting to trust that I might live a while longer than I expected. Fourteen years, beyond, in good health. What will I do with all that time? How will I ever be worthy of it?

On the subway ride home, there were delays on the F train and I had to get off and transfer to the C. I don't usually take the C train. The walk from the closest stop is still about half a mile from my apartment and less populated and on a darker street, so I avoid it. But that night, I had no choice. As I waited on the platform for the train, I tried to think of all the ways I could be better. I could go to the gym more; I could go to the gym at all. I could volunteer again at a hospital, the way I used to in high school. But I hated it then and I only did it as a way to spend time with a boy I had a crush on for about a decade. He wanted to volunteer at Children's Hospital, so I did, too, even though I spent plenty of time there already. As a patient, I hated volunteers—especially the woman and her Dalmatian who used to go from room to room dressed the same, asking if you needed a little love and remarking to me that a smile was really my best medicine. My mother would kindly usher her out of the room or lie and say I was allergic to dogs. I love dogs, which is why I think putting green glitter eye shadow and tutus on them is cruel. "You should tell her she can't come in because she's terrible," I would say, and my mother would laugh.

When I volunteered, nurses would send me into the rooms of patients who were younger than me and had similar heart conditions. Mostly, I would listen—to what they were afraid of, the worry about scarring, etc.—and nod my head. Kids don't talk about death much. They talk about maybe something going vaguely wrong during surgery or the scar they'll have when they wake up, but they don't talk about maybe not waking up. It's sweet, I think, because even in hospitals, most of them haven't learned death yet. I was careful not to say things like "Cheer up," or to beg for smiles, or to mention the gravity of any given situation. Sometimes we just played a board game and they'd ask me my age. Sixteen. And they'd ask me if I had a scar. Yes. And the girls would ask if they could see it. Sure. And the boys would ask if I knew how to drive. Yep. But it was hard for me to sit on that side of the bed knowing there was really no difference between us and though I'd been lucky thus far, my luck might slip out from under me at any time and then that damned lady with her Dalmatian would be there knocking on my door. So I asked the volunteer coordinator if I could be transferred to the Natal Intensive Care Unit. There, nobody needed my advice, and it was enough just to be comfortable around a lot of tubing and blood and to hold the babies whose parents couldn't be there to hold them all day as mine had. I could do that again, I thought as I boarded the C train. I could hold babies.

Before the transplant, my parents took me to see an abbot. They're both rabbis and my mother had a habit of taking me to every healer who rolled through town while I was growing up. Mostly, they didn't work, but sometimes we had miracles. The abbot was not a healer, though, my paents said; he was just a holy man. We sat in his office, my mother, father, and I. He asked me if I had any questions for him or for God.

I was tired. I had been waiting a year already and I was declining in health and sanity. I asked the abbot if it was okay not to know if I wanted the heart to come. I asked him if it was okay to sometimes smoke cigarettes in Vermont with my boyfriend, if I couldn't do that anymore when the new heart came because it wouldn't be mine to destroy, the way this one was. I asked him if it was okay that I had thought about it a great deal and I did not want to know the donor or think of them every day because I liked the person I was and I didn't want to risk losing myself to an organ. I asked him how I could deserve the heart better. I did not cry. My parents were quiet.

The abbot was soft-spoken. He wore wire-rimmed glasses and had white hair. He stayed still when he spoke, occasionally raising his hand to point to nothing in particular. "I think," he said, "that these are good questions. It's good to ask questions. But now that you've asked"—he raised his hand—"you can rest. You need a new heart, you'll get a new heart, and the hardest part, God willing, will be your waiting. So perhaps you give up. Give it all up to God."

The words we use to describe the sick, how we praise those who put on a brave face, how I received extra stickers and lollipops when I did not cry as a child, how we call people who don't complain "strong" and often compare illness to illness and then say, "It can always be worse." We demand gratitude. The abbot offered me a way out of that narrative, a silver branch to lift me out of the thinking that things could always be worse, a break from a crushing kind of gratitude. *Give up*. I imagined myself sinking to the bottom of a great body of water, not swimming, and not able to breathe until I reached the bottom.

The night before the call came, I sat in the passenger seat of Joey's green minivan, a defibrillator vest strapped to my chest and an IV in my arm. I cried so hard, I started to gag. "I want it so bad," I said. "I give up." She repeated it was coming over and over again as she rubbed the part of my back not taken up by the vest. My heart was beating very fast and there was a beeping from inside my bag—a warning that the vest would shock me in fifteen seconds if I did not press the right button on the battery pack because an arrhythmia might be pending. I dug around in my bag and could not find the battery.

"Adina, don't be funny. Adina, please, find that fucking battery."

"I'm trying." I laughed.

I found it with a few seconds to spare and the pack was quiet once again. I turned to Joey and apologized for scaring her.

I always thought dying would feel worse. I thought there would be more pain, I thought death would be clear. When the surgeons removed my old heart, they said I was lucky my liver wasn't failing, I was lucky to be alive; I couldn't have waited any longer. "Thank you," I said to everyone in the hospital that week I recovered. *Thank you, thank you, thank you*, compulsively, like a tic, until *thank you* was the only sound I made in exhalation before sleep.

125

It was nearly midnight when I stepped off the C train and started walking down the platform toward the Washington Avenue exit. I had my headphones in and I was listening to Otis Redding's "That's How Strong My Love Is" on repeat.

And there he was, the man from the bar, my heart twin; he was on the platform, heading toward the opposite exit, and hadn't seen me. We'd been on the same train, in different cars. Maybe it also took him an hour and a half to get home. I paused and recognized my choice—I could say something or not. I thought about what Joey said, about how maybe people don't think in terms of who is more or less traumatized, and how I can't know what his transplant was like but maybe it would give both of us something to hear him tell the story of it. So when I stepped off the train at a stop I don't usually go to and he was there, walking toward the exit, I rose up and took my luck's hand.

"Jesse!" I yelled. "Hey, Jesse!"

He turned around and we walked back toward each other. We met in the middle and I said, "I'm sorry for being so weird at the bar."

"Me, too," he said.

"It's just that it's not something I talk about in bars or otherwise. It's not something I usually share with people."

"Me, neither," he said.

"But you should know, it delighted me, and Joey, to hear fourteen years." We laughed a little, then hugged and said maybe we'd get coffee sometime and do it right. Then we parted ways.

Aboveground, I had missed calls from my dad and my mom. Now that I live in New York, we usually talk while I'm walking somewhere. I can still hear the delight in their voices when they ask, "What are you doing?" and I reply that I'm walking. I called my dad because he was more likely to be awake. He asked me where I was and I told him the whole story of the night—of the boy with fourteen years, of Joey, of the train delays and the subway stop I never go to. At the end, I said, "Sometimes the universe just shouts *I Got You*, y'know? And you feel right."

"Yeah," he said. "That's like God."

The Adina Talve-Goodman Fellowship

I FIRST MET ADINA in the summer of 2010, when she interned at *One Story*, the literary magazine I cofounded with Maribeth Batcha in Brooklyn. After a brief break, she returned to us, first as an assistant and later as *One Story*'s managing editor, beginning in March 2012. Adina quickly became a vibrant and vital member of our New York literary community. Those who interacted with her through *One Story*'s editorial department, writing classes, or public events, like our annual fundraiser, knew right away that she was special. She had a way of disarming—and charming—everyone. She filled *One Story*'s office with laughter, music, and joy.

Adina stepped into our lives during a window of stability, so while her health shaped the narrative of her life, it did not define her time with us. At *One Story*, she traveled to book festivals across the country, helped our nonprofit apply for grants, managed our volunteer readers, mentored dozens of interns, ran our summer writers' conference, perched on ladders while hanging decorations made from punctuation marks, ate a truckload of doughnuts, and tore up the dance floor whenever Robyn played.

Adina also spent many, many hours writing to emerging authors and encouraging their work. *One Story* publishes just twelve stories a year, which means we have to pass on a lot of manuscripts. Adina took the time to write personal, detailed letters to those submitters, speaking with care and kindness from one writer to another, creating her own (as one recipient called them) "antidotes to rejection." She had a strong interest in issues of embodied difference, illness, and suffering and helped *One Story* organize donations to prisons. Every day, she used her voice to amplify the voices of others. She had a knack for finding those who needed help and helping them, whenever and wherever they needed it.

In that same spirit of enthusiasm and advocacy, *One Story* now offers the Adina Talve-Goodman Fellowship. Founded with a generous donation from the Talve-Goodman family, this educational fellowship offers a yearlong mentorship on the craft of fiction writing with *One Story* magazine. It supports an early-career writer of fiction who has not yet published a book and whose work speaks to issues and experiences related to inhabiting bodies of difference. This means writing that centers, celebrates, or reclaims being marginalized through the lens of race, ethnicity, gender, sexuality, class, religion, illness, disability, trauma, migration, displacement, dispossession, or imprisonment. The fellow receives a stipend, a year of free writing classes offered by *One Story*, and a full manuscript review and consultation. Our hope is to give a writer outside the fold a significant boost in their career. Previous winners include Nay Saysourinho (2019), Arvin Ramgoolam (2020), Diana Veiga (2021), and Ani Cooney (2022). Adina was a lighthouse for her family, friends, and colleagues, and *One Story* is honored to be facilitating this fellowship with the Talve-Goodman family so that her love of storytelling and her vision for a better world can live on.

Not long after Adina joined us at *One Story*, I gave a public lecture on creating fictional characters. About fifty people came to listen. "Characters are a lot like superheroes," I said. "They need a costume, a backstory, a weakness, a mission, and a superpower." I asked for a volunteer to help me demonstrate, and Adina's hand shot up. She scampered to the front of the crowd and gamely put on a few superhero props that I'd brought: a blue mask, purple tights, a cape, a shield, and a plastic sword. She began to strike dramatic poses while people shouted out ideas for the character we were creating. I wish I'd written down all of the details of this improv, but the only thing I can remember now is this: Besides tremendous strength and the ability to fly, the audience decided that one of Adina's superpowers was smelling like lavender.

I'll never forget the look of complete delight on Adina's face when she was given this oddball ability. It was the same open-mouth grin and bright, wide eyes that shone in our office when she'd say, "Oh! Oh! What if we . . ." and then brought her fantastic imagination and brilliant, madcap clown energy into the room. To Adina, lavender was the *perfect* superpower, and she doubled down, declaring that her scent was so potent that she could use it to change people's moods—relax enemies into submission, or make a crowd of strangers feel loved and blissfully calm. Adina laughed and raised her plastic sword over her head. She hollered a battle cry: "*LAVENDER!*" And the audience went wild.

This was just one of many wild stunts that Adina helped us pull off at *One Story*. She spun her own particular brand of magic. Since she left us, I've been trying to do things that she would do—have more conversations with strangers, give money to street musicians, look out for my neighbors, speak more intimately and honestly to the people I love. In each of these small acts, I feel her beside me, just as she appears in the pages of this book: a hero in colorful scarves and overalls, with a backstory that inspires us to seize the day, a weakness for glitter and Cher, a mission of forgiveness and understanding, and a powerful, unforgettable heart that beats inside every word.

—Hannah Tinti

Biography

ADINA TALVE-GOODMAN was born on December 12, 1986. She was raised in St. Louis by her parents, Rabbi James Stone Goodman and Rabbi Susan Talve, along with her sister, Sarika Talve-Goodman, and her brother, Jacob Talve-Goodman. She attended Clayton High School and Washington University in St. Louis, where she studied Performance Studies, as well as Women, Gender, and Sexuality Studies. She became a well-known actress in the local theater scene, performed as a star clown in an Italian clown school, played King Lear at the London Globe, and started seriously pursuing creative writing. During this time, at nineteen years old, Adina received a heart transplant, due to a congenital heart condition, and began writing about it. After moving to Brooklyn in 2010, she joined the staff of the celebrated literary magazine *One Story*, and over the next six years, Adina poured her energy and enthusiasm into advocating for emerging writers, becoming a much-beloved member of the New York literary community. In 2015, she won the *Bellevue Literary Review*'s Nonfiction Prize with her essay "I Must Have Been That Man," and in 2016 she began attending the University of Iowa Nonfiction Writing Program. She was working on her first book when she was diagnosed with cancer. Adina passed away on January 12, 2018. This collection of essays is unfinished but full of truth and beauty. To read it is to hear her voice. We were so lucky to have known her.

Contributors
and Collaborators

Jo Firestone is a comedian whose work can be seen on *The Tonight Show Starring Jimmy Fallon*, *Joe Pera Talks with You*, *High Maintenance*, *Shrill*, and more. She can be heard on Maximum Fun's *Dr. Gameshow*, a podcast she cohosts with Manolo Moreno, and Comedy Central's *Everyday Decisions*, a podcast she hosts by herself. Her album, *The Hits*, is available on Comedy Central Records, and if you like puns, check out Punderdome: A Card Game for Pun Lovers. Her special, *Good Timing with Jo Firestone*, featuring sixteen senior citizens from her online comedy class, is out now on Peacock.

Rabbi James Stone Goodman is a writer and musician playing with hybrid forms. He earned his MFA in poetry from the University of Missouri-

St. Louis and studied classical Greek language and literature with Dr. George Carver at Arizona State University. He trained as a rabbi at Hebrew Union College and studied Classical Kabbalah with a manuscripts expert at the world-class Klau Library. He currently serves as a rabbi at Central Reform Congregation in St. Louis. Along with a small coalition of dedicated loyalists to the cause, Rabbi Jim has worked in addictions support, mental health, and prison outreach. He performs with several musical groups, and has recorded eleven CDs of original poetry, story, and music based on traditional forms. His writing has appeared in many publications, including the literary journal *Book of Matches*.

Rabbi Susan Talve is the founding rabbi of Central Reform Congregation, located within the city limits of St. Louis. When other congregations were leaving the city for the suburbs, Rabbi Susan joined with a small group to be on the front line of fighting the racism and poverty plaguing the urban center. Rabbi Susan has led her congregation in promoting radical hospitality and inclusivity by developing ongoing relationships with African American and Muslim congregations, and by fostering civil liberties for the LGBTQ community. Today CRC serves as a home to generations of LGBTQ families and to many Jews of color of all ages. She is the recipient of three honorary doctorates and numerous awards, and is the coauthor of two books and many published articles and stories. Most important, she is the spouse of Rabbi James Stone Goodman, the grateful mother of Jacob, Sarika, and Adina of blessed memory, and the grandmother of Harry and George.

Sarika Talve-Goodman, MS, LMSW, PhD, (she/her), is a literary scholar and somatic psychotherapist. She received her MS in Narrative Medicine from Columbia University and her doctorate in literature from the University of California, San Diego, specializing in modernism studies, disability studies, trauma theory, Jewish cultural studies, and critical theories of race, gender, and sexuality. She has researched and taught at the Hebrew University in Jerusalem and Oberlin College. When Adina became ill and died, Sarika left Oberlin and paused her academic career to be with her family. She is currently a full-time clinician, training as an integrative trauma therapist in St. Louis.

Hannah Tinti is a writer, editor, and teacher. Her best-selling novel *The Good Thief* won The Center for Fiction First Novel Prize, and her story collection, *Animal Crackers*, was a runner-up for the PEN/Hemingway Award. Her novel *The Twelve Lives of Samuel Hawley* is a national best-seller and is being developed for television with Netflix. She teaches creative writing at New York University's MFA program and cofounded the Sirenland Writers Conference. Tinti is also the cofounder and executive editor of *One Story* magazine, which won the AWP Small Press Publisher Award, CLMP's Firecracker Award, a 2020 Whiting Prize, and the PEN/Nora Magid Award for Magazine Editing.